SINGLE MOM'S PREGNANCY GUIDE

A Comprehensive Pregnancy Guide For Single Mothers

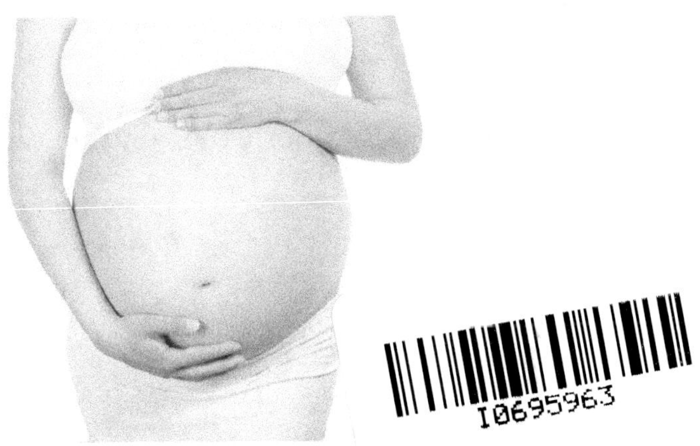

Kimberley A. Garcia

Table Of Contents

INTRODUCTION

Chapter 1

Chapter 2

Chapter 3

Chapter 4

Chapter 5

Chapter 6

INTRODUCTION

Congratulations on taking this incredible step into motherhood! The path you're embarking upon as a single mom-to-be is both inspiring and full of unique challenges and joys. This book,"**Single Mom**'s **Pregnancy Guide**," is here to offer you guidance, support, and empowerment throughout your pregnancy journey and beyond.

Becoming a mother is a transformative experience, and doing so as a single mom adds an extra layer of strength to your story. You might be feeling a mixture of excitement, anticipation, and perhaps even some apprehension. Rest assured, you are not alone in this journey. Countless women before you have navigated the path of single motherhood during pregnancy and beyond, and their experiences can offer you insights, wisdom, and solidarity.

In this **guide**, we'll walk with you through each trimester, addressing the physical, emotional, and practical aspects of your pregnancy. From deciding to embark on this journey, to nurturing your newborn, and navigating the complexities of postpartum life, we're here to provide you with knowledge, tools, and strategies to make your journey as smooth as possible.

You'll find information on prenatal care, self-care, legal considerations, and creating a support network that empowers you. We'll also delve into topics such as maintaining your emotional well-being, building connections with other single moms, and finding the resources you need to thrive.

Remember, being a single mom doesn't mean you're alone. You have within you a wellspring of strength and resilience that will carry you through the challenges and help you savor the joyful moments. This book is your companion, your guide, and your source of reassurance. Each chapter is designed to uplift you, provide you with practical advice, and remind you that you are capable of embracing your journey with grace and determination.

As you turn the **pages** of this **guide**, let each word remind you that you are part of a community of strong, nurturing, and empowered single moms who have come before you and who stand beside you. Your journey into motherhood is a story worth celebrating, and we are honored to be a part of it.

Get ready to embark on this remarkable journey of self-discovery, growth, and boundless love. You've got this, and we're here to support you every step of the way.

Embracing Your Journey As A Single Mom-To-Be

Becoming a single mom-to-be is a unique and courageous journey that comes with its own set of challenges and rewards. While it may seem daunting, embracing this journey can lead to personal growth, empowerment, and a deep connection with both yourself and your future child. This guide also aims to provide insights and guidance on how to navigate this path with grace, positivity, and confidence.

Embrace Self-Care:
Taking care of yourself is paramount during this journey. Prioritize your physical, emotional, and mental well-being through regular exercise, proper nutrition, and relaxation techniques. Engage in activities that bring you joy and help alleviate stress. Remember that your well-being directly impacts your baby's well-being.

Build a Support System:
Surround yourself with a supportive network of friends, family, and possibly a single-parent community. Lean on them for emotional support, practical advice, and assistance when needed. Sharing your feelings and experiences can help reduce feelings of isolation and create a sense of belonging.

Cultivate a Positive Mindset:
Approach your journey with a positive outlook. Focus on the exciting aspects of becoming a mother, rather than dwelling on the challenges. Practice gratitude daily and remind yourself of your strengths and capabilities. A positive mindset can help you overcome obstacles and create a nurturing environment for yourself and your child.

Financial Planning:
As a single mom-to-be, financial planning becomes crucial. Create a budget that covers prenatal care, baby essentials, and future expenses. Research available resources such as government assistance programs, grants, and local support services that can provide financial aid and guidance.

Prepare for Parenthood:
Educate yourself about pregnancy, childbirth, and parenting. Attend prenatal classes, read books, and seek advice from experienced parents. Developing a strong foundation of

knowledge will help you approach motherhood with confidence and reduce uncertainties.

Nurture Self-Identity:
While embracing the role of a single mom-to-be, remember to preserve your individuality. Pursue your passions, interests, and career goals, adjusting them as necessary to accommodate your new responsibilities. Maintaining your sense of self will contribute to your overall happiness and well-rounded parenting.

Effective Time Management:
Balancing work, personal life, and impending motherhood requires effective time management. Prioritize tasks, delegate when possible, and create a flexible schedule that allows you to meet your responsibilities while also dedicating quality time to yourself and your child.

Seek Professional Guidance:
Therapists, counselors, and support groups specializing in single parenting can offer valuable insights and coping strategies.

Professional guidance can help you address any emotional challenges, anxiety, or stress that may arise during your journey.

Embrace Imperfections:
Perfection is unattainable, and it's okay to make mistakes. Embrace the imperfections and understand that learning and growth come from these experiences. Be patient with yourself and celebrate the small victories along the way.

Embracing your journey as a single mom-to-be is an empowering and transformative experience. By prioritizing self-care, building a strong support system, maintaining a positive mindset, and seeking knowledge, you can navigate this path with confidence and grace. Remember that every step you take brings you closer to creating a loving and nurturing environment for yourself and your future child. Your journey is a testament to your strength, resilience, and unwavering love.

Chapter 1

Health And Lifestyle Adjustments

In this chapter, we'll explore essential tips and suggestions to help you prioritize your well-being and that of your growing baby.

Nutrition and Diet:
Emphasize a balanced diet rich in fruits, vegetables, lean proteins, whole grains, and dairy products.
Consume prenatal vitamins as recommended by your healthcare provider.
Stay hydrated by drinking plenty of water throughout the day.

Regular Prenatal Care:
Schedule regular appointments with an obstetrician or midwife to monitor the health of both you and your baby.

Follow the recommended prenatal screening and tests to ensure the well-being of your child.

Physical Activity:
Engage in safe and gentle exercises like walking, swimming, and prenatal yoga to maintain physical fitness and alleviate discomfort.
Consult your healthcare provider before starting any new exercise routine.

Stress Management:
Practice relaxation techniques such as deep breathing, meditation, and mindfulness to reduce stress levels.
Seek emotional support from friends, family, or support groups to share your feelings and concerns.

Sleep and Rest:
Prioritize getting enough sleep and rest to support your energy levels and overall health.
Consider using supportive pillows to help you find a comfortable sleeping position as your pregnancy progresses.

Time Management:
Plan your daily activities and responsibilities to avoid unnecessary stress.
Delegate tasks when possible and don't hesitate to ask for help when needed.

Financial Planning:
Create a budget to manage expenses related to prenatal care, childbirth, and baby essentials.
Look into available government programs or community resources that can provide financial assistance.

Emotional Well-being:
Allow yourself to experience a range of emotions and seek professional counseling if needed.
Engage in activities that bring you joy and relaxation, whether it's reading, listening to music, or pursuing a hobby.

Bonding with Your Baby:

Talk, sing, and read to your baby to foster early bonding.

Consider joining prenatal classes or workshops to learn about baby care and parenting.

Birth Planning:

Create a birth plan that outlines your preferences for labor, delivery, and postpartum care.

Identify a support person or doula to be by your side during labor if desired.

Pregnancy is a transformative time, and being a single mom adds unique dimensions to the experience. By prioritizing your health, seeking support, and making thoughtful lifestyle adjustments, you can navigate this journey with confidence and create a nurturing environment for both you and your baby. Remember, you're not alone, and there are resources available to help you every step of the way.

Navigating The First Trimester

The first trimester, spanning from weeks 1 to 12, is a critical phase filled with physical and emotional changes. Successfully navigating this period requires careful planning, self-care, and a strong support system. Here's a comprehensive guide to help you thrive during the first trimester of pregnancy:

1. **Confirming Pregnancy and Medical Care**:
The first step is confirming the pregnancy through a home pregnancy test or a visit to a healthcare provider. Early prenatal care is vital for assessing the health of both the mother and the developing fetus. Establishing a relationship with a healthcare provider will ensure proper monitoring and guidance throughout the pregnancy.

2. **Emotional Well-being**:
Coping with the emotional changes during the first trimester is crucial. Hormonal shifts can lead to mood swings and anxiety. Engaging in relaxation techniques such as meditation, deep breathing, and gentle exercise can help manage

stress. Connecting with other single moms or joining support groups can provide a sense of community and understanding.

3. Nutrition and Hydration:

A balanced diet rich in essential nutrients is essential for the well-being of both the mother and the baby. Folic acid, iron, calcium, and protein are particularly important during this stage. Consultation with a healthcare provider or a registered dietitian can help tailor a nutrition plan to meet individual needs. Staying hydrated is equally important.

4. Managing Morning Sickness:

Morning sickness, characterized by nausea and vomiting, is a common symptom during the first trimester. Eating small, frequent meals and avoiding trigger foods can help alleviate these symptoms. Ginger, acupressure bands, and prescribed medications can also provide relief.

5. Work and Lifestyle Adjustments:

Single moms may need to evaluate their work situations and lifestyle choices. If feasible, consider discussing flexible work arrangements with your employer to accommodate medical appointments and potential fatigue. Avoiding alcohol, tobacco, and certain medications is essential for the baby's health.

6. **Building a Support System**:
Enlist the support of family, friends, and healthcare professionals. Communicate your needs and concerns to your support network, as they can offer assistance with daily tasks, emotional support, and advice. If possible, establish a birthing plan that outlines who will be present during labor and delivery.

7. **Financial Planning**:
Financial planning is a crucial aspect of single parenthood. Research available resources, such as government programs, community services, and financial assistance options. Budgeting for medical expenses, baby essentials, and maternity leave is essential to alleviate stress later on.

8. **Preparing for Parenthood**:
Use the first trimester to educate yourself about pregnancy, childbirth, and parenting. Attend prenatal classes, read books, and explore online resources to gain knowledge and build confidence. Making informed decisions about childbirth options, breastfeeding, and baby care will help ease anxieties.

9. **Self-Care**:
Taking care of oneself is paramount. Ensure you get adequate rest, engage in moderate exercise, and prioritize activities that bring joy and relaxation. Pamper yourself occasionally to maintain a positive outlook and a strong mental state.

10. **Monitoring Health**:
Regular prenatal check-ups and screenings are vital to track the baby's development and the mother's health. Any unusual symptoms, bleeding, or severe pain should be immediately reported to a healthcare provider.

Navigating the first trimester of pregnancy as a single mom is undoubtedly a challenge, but with careful planning, self-care, and a strong support network, it is a journey that can be embraced with optimism. Remember, seeking help when needed and staying informed are key to ensuring a healthy pregnancy and laying the foundation for a fulfilling parenting journey ahead.

Chapter 2

<u>Dealing With Morning Sickness And Fatigue</u>

Dealing with morning sickness and fatigue during this time can be especially daunting. However, with the right strategies and support in place, single moms can successfully manage these symptoms and prioritize their well-being and the health of their babies.

Understanding Morning Sickness:
Morning sickness, characterized by nausea and vomiting, is a common pregnancy symptom. Contrary to its name, it can occur at any time of the day. To manage morning sickness effectively, single mothers can:

1. Eat Small, Frequent Meals: Consuming small, nutrient-rich meals throughout the

day can help stabilize blood sugar levels and alleviate nausea.

2. Stay Hydrated: Sipping water or clear fluids can prevent dehydration, a common trigger for nausea.

3. Ginger and Lemon: Incorporating ginger or lemon into meals or drinks has been known to ease nausea for some pregnant women.

4. Avoid Triggers: Identifying and avoiding triggers such as strong odors or certain foods can help prevent bouts of nausea.

Managing Fatigue:
Pregnancy-related fatigue is often attributed to hormonal changes and increased energy demands on the body. Single moms can combat fatigue by:

1. Prioritizing Sleep: Establishing a consistent sleep schedule and creating a

comfortable sleep environment can improve the quality and duration of sleep.

2. Asking for Help: Enlisting the support of friends, family, or a babysitter can provide essential breaks and rest periods.

3. Napping: Short naps during the day can help replenish energy levels, but avoiding long naps close to bedtime is recommended.

4. Gentle Exercise: Engaging in light physical activities, such as walking or prenatal yoga, can boost energy and alleviate fatigue.

Seeking Emotional Support:
Dealing with pregnancy symptoms alone can be emotionally challenging. Single mothers can benefit from seeking emotional support through:

1. Support Groups: Connecting with other single pregnant women can provide a

sense of camaraderie and a platform to share experiences.

2. Counseling or Therapy: Speaking with a professional can help manage stress, anxiety, and any emotional toll that pregnancy symptoms may bring.

3. Open Communication: Talking to close friends, family, or a trusted confidant about struggles and needs can alleviate feelings of isolation.

4. Online Communities: Participating in online forums or social media groups dedicated to pregnancy can offer a virtual support network.

Being a single mom while dealing with morning sickness and fatigue during pregnancy is undoubtedly a challenge, but it's important to remember that seeking help, implementing practical strategies, and prioritizing self-care can make a significant difference. By taking care

By taking care of your physical and emotional well-being, you can lay the foundation for a healthier, more manageable pregnancy journey for yourself and your growing baby.

<u>Blossoming Through The Second Trimester</u>

The second trimester, spanning from weeks 13 to 27, is often referred to as the "honeymoon phase" of pregnancy. During this time, women experience physical and emotional changes, which can be uniquely challenging for single mothers navigating pregnancy alone. Let's explore how pregnant single moms can blossom through the second trimester, embracing both the joys and hurdles.

Embracing Physical Changes:
The second trimester is marked by noticeable physical changes, such as a growing belly and increased energy levels. For single mothers,

these changes can be a source of empowerment, serving as a visual reminder of the strength required to nurture new life. As the body adapts, pregnant single moms need to prioritize self-care, including proper nutrition, regular exercise, and sufficient rest.

Navigating Emotional Well-being:
Emotional well-being is crucial during pregnancy, especially for single mothers who may experience feelings of isolation or anxiety. The second trimester often brings relief from early pregnancy symptoms and a surge of maternal hormones. Single moms can capitalize on this period to engage in activities that bring joy and emotional balance. Connecting with support networks, seeking counseling, or joining pregnancy groups can provide a sense of community and understanding.

Building a Support System:
While every pregnancy journey is unique, building a robust support system is particularly important for single moms. The second trimester

is an opportune time to identify and connect with friends, family, or support groups that can offer practical assistance and emotional encouragement. Single mothers can also explore resources available in their communities, such as parenting classes or financial aid programs.

Planning for the Future:
The middle trimester offers a window of opportunity for pregnant single mothers to plan for the future. This includes decisions about birthing options, potential childcare arrangements, and postpartum plans. By addressing these aspects during the second trimester, single moms can approach the third trimester with a greater sense of preparedness and reduced stress.

Celebrating Milestones:
Amid the challenges, pregnant single moms need to celebrate the milestones of their journey. The second trimester is often when the baby's gender is revealed, creating an exciting moment for both the mother and her support network. Hosting a

small gender reveal event or participating in pregnancy photoshoots can infuse moments of joy and positivity into the journey.

Blossoming through the second trimester as a pregnant single mom is a testament to strength, determination, and resilience. By embracing the physical changes, nurturing emotional well-being, building a support system, planning for the future, and celebrating milestones, single mothers can navigate this phase with grace and positivity. The journey is a reminder that, despite the challenges, the love and dedication of a mother know no bounds, and the second trimester marks a significant step towards welcoming a new life into the world.

Chapter 3

Navigating Body Changes and Prioritizing Self-Care During Pregnancy

In this chapter, we will be exploring the body changes experienced during pregnancy and emphasizing the importance of self-care for single mothers during this crucial period.

Body Changes During Pregnancy:

1. Weight Gain: Single mothers experience weight gain as a natural part of pregnancy. This is due to the growth of the fetus, increased blood volume, and changes in hormone levels. Embracing this change and maintaining a balanced diet are essential for both the mother's and baby's well-being.

2. Skin Changes: Hormonal fluctuations may lead to various skin changes, such as stretch marks, pigmentation changes, and acne. Embracing these changes as part of the pregnancy journey and using suitable skincare products can help manage skin concerns.

3. Breast Changes: Breasts undergo significant changes, becoming larger and more sensitive as they prepare for breastfeeding. Investing in comfortable maternity bras and practicing breast care can help manage discomfort.

4. Muscle and Joint Changes: As the body prepares for childbirth, ligaments loosen, potentially leading to joint pain. Engaging in low-impact exercises and practicing gentle stretches can provide relief and maintain flexibility.

5. Digestive Changes: Hormonal changes can slow down digestion, leading to

constipation and heartburn. Staying hydrated, consuming fiber-rich foods, and eating smaller, frequent meals can help manage these digestive changes.

Self-Care for Single Mothers During Pregnancy:

1. Prioritize Rest: Single mothers often juggle multiple responsibilities. Prioritizing adequate rest and sleep is crucial for maintaining energy levels and promoting overall well-being.

2. Seek Support: Reach out to friends, family, and support groups for emotional and practical assistance. Accepting help with daily tasks can ease the physical strain on your body.

3. Nutrition: Maintain a balanced diet rich in nutrients, vitamins, and minerals essential for both your health and the baby's development. Consult a healthcare

provider for personalized dietary recommendations.

4. Exercise: Engage in gentle exercises approved by your healthcare provider. Prenatal yoga, swimming, and walking can help improve circulation, alleviate discomfort, and reduce stress.

5. Mindfulness and Relaxation: Practice techniques like meditation, deep breathing, and prenatal massages to manage stress, anxiety, and mood swings.

6. Regular Check-ups: Attend scheduled prenatal appointments to monitor your health and the baby's progress. Openly discuss any concerns with your healthcare provider.

7. Bonding Time: Allocate time to bond with your growing baby. Talking, singing, and playing soothing music can create a sense of connection.

8. Educate Yourself: Stay informed about the different stages of pregnancy and childbirth. Knowledge empowers you to make informed decisions about your health and birth preferences.

Embracing body changes and practicing self-care can positively impact both your physical and emotional well-being. Remember that seeking help, nurturing your body, and prioritizing self-care are essential steps in ensuring a healthy and fulfilling pregnancy journey as a single mom.

Legal And Custodial Considerations

Bringing a child into the world is a monumental journey, especially when undertaken as a single mother. Beyond the physical and emotional aspects, there are legal and custodial considerations that demand attention. Let's delve into the crucial facets of legal and custodial matters that single mothers should be aware of during pregnancy and beyond.

Legal Considerations:

Parental Rights and Responsibilities:
As a single mother, it's important to understand your legal rights and responsibilities as a parent. Establishing legal paternity, if necessary, ensures that the other parent shares responsibilities, including financial support and decision-making.

Custody Arrangements:
Exploring custody options early on can help prevent conflicts down the road. Depending on your circumstances, you might consider sole custody, joint custody, or visitation rights for the other parent.

Child Support:
Single mothers have the right to seek financial support from the child's other parent. Child support orders are usually determined based on factors such as income and the child's needs.

Estate Planning:
Drafting a will is vital to secure your child's future. It allows you to designate a guardian for your child in case of unforeseen circumstances and ensures that your child inherits your assets.

Custodial Considerations:

Prenatal Care:
Prioritize prenatal health for both yourself and your baby. Regular medical check-ups, proper nutrition, and a healthy lifestyle are essential for a successful pregnancy.

Support System:
Building a strong support network of family, friends, and support groups can provide emotional and practical assistance throughout your pregnancy and beyond.

Maternity Leave and Employment Rights:
Familiarize yourself with maternity leave policies in your region. Know your rights

regarding time off work, job security, and possible accommodations during pregnancy and postpartum.

Postpartum Planning:
Anticipate the challenges of postpartum recovery and childcare. Consider arrangements for childcare, flexible work options, and any necessary medical care.

Embarking on the journey of pregnancy as a single mother requires careful consideration of legal and custodial aspects. By being informed about your rights, responsibilities, and available resources, you can ensure a smoother transition into motherhood. Remember that seeking legal advice, building a strong support system, and prioritizing your child's well-being will empower you to navigate these considerations with confidence.

Thriving In The Third Trimester

For a single mother-to-be, the third trimester can be both physically demanding and emotionally overwhelming. Navigating this crucial phase requires a combination of self-care, support systems, and practical strategies to ensure not only the well-being of the mother but also the healthy development of the unborn child. In this write-up, we will explore valuable insights and tips for single mothers to thrive during the third trimester of pregnancy.

Prioritizing Self-Care:
1. Adequate Rest: As the body undergoes significant changes, rest becomes essential. Prioritize sleep by creating a comfortable sleeping environment and establishing a regular sleep schedule.
2. Nutritious Diet: A balanced diet rich in vitamins, minerals, and proteins is crucial for both the mother's and the baby's development. Consult a healthcare provider for dietary recommendations.
3. Gentle Exercise: Engaging in light exercises, such as prenatal yoga or

walking, can alleviate discomfort and boost energy levels. Always consult a healthcare provider before starting any exercise routine.

Building a Support Network:
1. Reach Out to Loved Ones: Share your feelings and concerns with friends and family who can provide emotional support and practical assistance.
2. Join Support Groups: Participate in local or online support groups for single mothers or expectant mothers to connect with individuals who are experiencing similar challenges.

Seeking Medical Care:
1. Regular Check-ups: Attend all prenatal appointments and follow medical advice to monitor both your health and the baby's progress.
2. Birth Plan: Discuss your birth plan with your healthcare provider and, if desired, choose a labor companion who can

provide physical and emotional support during labor.

Practical Preparation:

1. Baby Essentials: Prepare the necessary baby essentials, such as clothing, diapers, and a safe sleeping environment.
2. Childcare Arrangements: Research and plan for childcare options that suit your needs once the baby arrives.

Emotional Well-being:

1. Positive Mindset: Cultivate a positive outlook on your journey. Practicing mindfulness and relaxation techniques can help manage stress and anxiety.
2. Seek Professional Help: If you find yourself struggling emotionally, don't hesitate to seek counseling or therapy to address your feelings and concerns.

Time Management:

1. Create a Schedule: Organize your daily routine to balance work, prenatal

appointments, rest, and personal time. Utilize tools like calendars and reminders to stay on track.
2. Delegate Responsibilities: Don't hesitate to ask for help from friends, family, or even hired services to manage tasks that become challenging during pregnancy.

Thriving in the third trimester as a pregnant single mom is a combination of self-care, seeking support, and practical planning. By prioritizing your well-being, building a strong support network, and addressing both physical and emotional needs, you can navigate this phase with confidence and grace. Remember, you have the strength within you to embrace motherhood and provide a nurturing environment for your baby's growth and development.

Chapter 4

Preparing For Labor And Delivery

Preparing for labor and delivery is an important aspect of pregnancy, and for single mothers, the journey can come with its own set of challenges. While the process may seem daunting, with proper planning, support, and self-care, single mothers can navigate this phase with confidence and resilience. This chapter offers valuable insights and practical tips to help pregnant single moms prepare for labor and delivery.

Prenatal Care:
1. Seek regular prenatal medical care: Schedule and attend all prenatal appointments to monitor your health and the baby's development.
2. Choose a healthcare provider: Select a healthcare professional who understands

your circumstances and can provide appropriate guidance and support.
3. Attend childbirth education classes: These classes provide valuable information about labor, delivery, and postpartum care.

Build a Support System:
1. Reach out to family and friends: Lean on your support network for emotional and practical assistance during pregnancy, labor, and postpartum.
2. Consider a doula: A doula can provide continuous emotional and physical support during labor and delivery, enhancing your experience.

Create a Birth Plan:
1. Outline your preferences: Consider your preferences for pain management, medical interventions, and the atmosphere you want during labor.
2. Be flexible: Understand that birth plans may need adjustments, but having a

general guideline can help you feel more prepared.

Pack Your Hospital Bag:
1. Essentials for you: Include comfortable clothing, toiletries, snacks, important documents, and items that provide comfort.
2. Essentials for baby: Pack clothes, diapers, blankets, and other essentials for the baby's first moments.

Financial and Practical Preparations:
1. Budgeting: Plan for medical costs, postpartum expenses, and baby supplies. Look into available financial resources and assistance programs.
2. Arrange transportation: Ensure you have a reliable mode of transportation to the hospital when the time comes.

Emotional Well-being:
1. Seek counseling or therapy: Managing emotions during pregnancy can be

overwhelming. Professional help can provide coping strategies.
2. Practice mindfulness: Techniques such as meditation, deep breathing, and yoga can help manage stress and anxiety.

Postpartum Planning:
1. Arrange postpartum support: Line up help after the birth, whether from friends, family, or hired assistance.
2. Explore childcare options: Research daycare facilities or nannies if you need to return to work soon after childbirth.

Childbirth Education:
1. Educate yourself: Learn about the stages of labor, breathing techniques, and pain management options.
2. Attend parenting classes: These classes can equip you with essential skills for newborn care and breastfeeding.

Preparing for labor and delivery as a pregnant single mom involves a combination of practical preparation, emotional well-being, and building a strong support network. While the journey may have its challenges, with careful planning, open communication with healthcare professionals, and a positive mindset, you can approach childbirth with confidence and optimism. Remember that you are not alone, and there are resources and people available to help you every step of the way.

Welcoming Your Baby

Welcoming a new baby is a joyous and life-changing experience, but it can also be quite challenging, especially for single mothers. As a single mom, you are faced with unique circumstances that require careful planning, emotional resilience, and a strong support network. In this section, we will provide valuable insights and practical advice for single mothers as they embark on the journey of welcoming their precious bundle of joy.

I. **Emotional Preparation**:

1. Embrace the Journey: Emotionally prepare yourself for the arrival of your baby by acknowledging both the excitement and the challenges that lie ahead. Seek positive affirmations and connect with other single mothers for encouragement.

2. Self-Care: Prioritize self-care to maintain your emotional well-being. This includes getting enough rest, engaging in activities you love, and seeking therapy or counseling if needed.

II. **Financial Planning**:

1. Budgeting: Create a detailed budget that takes into account your current and anticipated expenses. Factor in costs like medical bills, baby essentials, daycare, and more.

2. Savings: Start building an emergency fund to provide a safety net in case unexpected expenses arise. Research government assistance programs and community resources that might offer financial support.

III. **Practical Preparation**:

1. Baby Essentials: Compile a list of essential items your baby will need, such as diapers, clothing, a crib, bottles, and formula if necessary. Look for secondhand items or ask friends and family for hand-me-downs to save money.

2. Childcare: Explore your options for childcare, whether it's daycare, hiring a nanny, or relying on family members. Plan to ensure you have a reliable and safe arrangement for when you return to work.

IV. **Building a Support Network**:

1. Family and Friends: Reach out to your family and friends for emotional support and practical help. They can assist with tasks like babysitting, meal preparation, and running errands.

2. Single Parent Groups: Join local or online support groups for single parents. These communities can offer advice, camaraderie, and a sense of belonging.

V. **Time Management**:

1. Prioritization: Learn to manage your time efficiently by prioritizing tasks and setting realistic expectations. Delegate when possible, and don't be afraid to ask for help.

2. Flexible Schedules: If your job allows, explore flexible work arrangements such as remote work or adjusted hours to accommodate your baby's needs.

VI. **Self-Development**:

1. Pursue Goals: While being a single mom is a significant responsibility, it's important to continue pursuing your personal and professional goals. Set small milestones and celebrate your achievements.

2. Continuous Learning: Equip yourself with parenting knowledge by reading books, attending workshops, and seeking advice from experienced parents.

Welcoming a baby as a single mom is undoubtedly a unique journey that requires careful planning, emotional resilience, and a strong support network. By preparing emotionally, financially, and practically, you can navigate this exciting chapter with confidence. Remember that you are not alone—there are resources, communities, and individuals ready to offer guidance and encouragement every step of the way.

Chapter 5

Balancing Single Parenthood And Self-Care

Single parenthood brings with it a unique set of challenges and responsibilities, and single moms often find themselves juggling the demands of parenting while trying to prioritize their well-being. Balancing single parenthood and self-care is essential for maintaining physical, emotional, and mental health. This chapter delves into practical strategies and insights to help single moms effectively manage their roles as caregivers while ensuring they don't neglect their self-care needs.

The Importance of Self-Care:
Self-care is not selfish: it is a fundamental aspect of maintaining a healthy and fulfilling life. Single moms can only provide the best for their children when they themselves are well-cared

for. Self-care encompasses various dimensions, including physical, emotional, mental, and social well-being.

Strategies for Balancing Single Parenthood and Self-Care:
   a. Establishing a Routine: Creating a structured daily routine helps single moms manage their time efficiently, ensuring they allocate time for both parenting responsibilities and self-care activities.
   b. Seeking Support: Building a network of friends, family members, or support groups can provide invaluable assistance and a much-needed emotional outlet.
   c. Time Management: Learning to prioritize tasks, delegate responsibilities, and utilize time-management tools can help single moms find time for self-care amidst their busy schedules.
   d. Setting Boundaries: Setting boundaries at work, with family, and in personal relationships prevents burnout and creates space for self-care.

e. Outsourcing When Possible: It's okay to ask for help or hire assistance for tasks like house cleaning or childcare to free up time for relaxation and self-care.

Self-Care Practices for Single Moms:

a. Physical Well-being: Regular exercise, a balanced diet, and adequate sleep contribute to improved energy levels and overall health.

b. Emotional Well-being: Engaging in activities that bring joy, practicing mindfulness, and seeking therapy can help manage stress and emotional challenges.

c. Mental Well-being: Pursuing hobbies, reading, or learning new skills stimulates the mind and provides a sense of accomplishment beyond parenting.

d. Social Well-Being: Nurturing social connections through friendships, community involvement, or online support groups combats feelings of isolation.

e. Alone Time: Taking short breaks for solitude, relaxation, or pursuing personal interests helps single moms recharge.

Overcoming Guilt and Prioritizing Self-Care:
a. Recognizing Guilt: Single moms often experience guilt when prioritizing themselves, but understanding that self-care enhances their ability to parent effectively can alleviate these feelings.
b. Lead by Example: Demonstrating the importance of self-care to children teaches them about healthy habits and self-respect.

Self-Care as a Long-Term Investment:
a. Sustainable Habits: Single moms should view self-care as an ongoing commitment rather than an occasional indulgence.
b. Modeling Healthy Relationships: By valuing their well-being, single moms set an example for their children about what it means to have a balanced and fulfilling life.

Balancing single parenthood and self-care is an intricate journey that requires intentionality and effort. By recognizing that self-care is not a luxury but a necessity, single moms can create healthier, more fulfilling lives for themselves and their children. Embracing self-care as an essential aspect of parenting ultimately leads to improved well-being, increased resilience, and a stronger foundation upon which to raise children.

Nurturing Postpartum Health and Wellness: A Guide for Single Moms

The journey of motherhood is a transformative experience that brings immense joy and challenges. For single mothers, navigating the postpartum period can be particularly demanding as they balance the responsibilities of parenthood with their own well-being. Postpartum health and wellness are crucial aspects that require attention and care to ensure both the mother and the baby thrive during this pivotal time.

I. **Physical Well-being**:

A. Rest and Sleep:

Prioritize sleep when the baby sleeps to combat fatigue.

Seek help from friends or family to share nighttime responsibilities.

B. Nutritional Needs:

Focus on a balanced diet rich in fruits, vegetables, whole grains, and lean proteins.

Consider meal prepping or using meal delivery services to save time.

C. Exercise:

Engage in light exercises, like walking or yoga, after consulting a healthcare professional.

Incorporate baby-friendly exercises to bond with your child while staying active.

II. **Emotional Well-being**:

A. Seek Support:

Build a support network of friends, family, and support groups.

Connect with other single moms to share experiences and advice.

B. Mental Health:

Monitor for signs of postpartum depression or anxiety and seek professional help if needed.

Practice mindfulness, deep breathing, and meditation to manage stress.

C. Self-Care:

Set aside time for self-care activities that rejuvenate your spirit.

Engage in hobbies and activities that bring joy and relaxation.

III. **Financial Wellness**:

A. Budgeting:

Create a budget that considers the additional expenses of raising a child.

Explore government assistance programs and community resources for financial support.

B. Career and Work-life Balance:

Explore flexible work options or remote work if possible.

Communicate openly with your employer about your needs as a single parent.

IV. **Social Well-being**:

A. Social Connections:

Foster friendships with other parents to combat feelings of isolation.

Attend parenting classes or playgroups to engage with other caregivers.

B. Dating and Relationships:

Take your time before introducing a new partner to your child.

Prioritize open communication with potential partners about your responsibilities.

V. **Child's Well-being**:

A. Bonding:

Establish a strong bond with your child through physical touch, eye contact, and nurturing activities.

Engage in regular playtime to promote cognitive and emotional development.

B. Childcare:

Explore reliable childcare options when you need time for personal activities or work.

Research and select caregivers carefully to ensure your child's safety and well-being.

As a single mom, your well-being is essential for providing the best possible care for your child. Prioritizing postpartum health involves a holistic approach that encompasses physical, emotional, financial, and social aspects. Remember that seeking support, practicing self-care, and nurturing your own growth are not only beneficial for you but also contribute to the overall happiness and success of your parenting journey.

Chapter 6

Thriving As A Single Mom

Being a single mom comes with its own set of challenges, but it is also a journey filled with empowerment, growth, and the potential for a thriving life. In today's world, more and more women are embracing the role of single mothers and demonstrating remarkable resilience and success. Let's delve into the strategies, mindset shifts, and support systems that contribute to the thriving of single moms.

Embracing Self-Care:
Single moms often find themselves juggling multiple responsibilities, leaving little time for themselves. Prioritizing self-care is essential for physical and mental well-being. Regular exercise, proper nutrition, adequate sleep, and activities that bring joy and relaxation can help

single moms recharge and maintain their resilience.

Building a Support Network:
Creating a strong support system is crucial. Single moms can reach out to family, friends, support groups, and online communities to connect with others who understand their experiences. Networking provides emotional support, practical advice, and a sense of belonging, reducing feelings of isolation.

Balancing Work and Parenting:
Achieving a balance between work and parenting is a common concern. Flexible work arrangements, effective time management, and setting clear boundaries can help single moms fulfill both their professional and parental responsibilities without burnout.

Financial Independence:
Single moms often handle the family's finances on their own. Creating a budget, setting financial goals, and seeking out resources for financial

assistance or education can empower single moms to take control of their financial future and provide for their families.

Pursuing Education and Career Goals:
Continuing education or pursuing career aspirations might seem challenging, but it's not impossible. Single moms can explore online courses, part-time education, or remote work opportunities that provide the flexibility needed to upgrade skills and advance in their careers.

Effective Co-Parenting:
In cases where co-parenting is possible, maintaining open communication and a cooperative approach is essential for the well-being of the children. Setting aside personal differences and focusing on the best interests of the child fosters a positive co-parenting environment.

Role Modeling and Empowering Children:
Single moms have the opportunity to be powerful role models for their children. By

demonstrating resilience, determination, and a positive attitude, they teach their children valuable life skills and the importance of overcoming challenges.

Time Management and Organization:
Single moms often have to manage a multitude of tasks simultaneously. Effective time management and organization skills can help them streamline tasks, reduce stress, and create more quality time to spend with their children.

Cultivating a Growth Mindset:
Adopting a growth mindset involves viewing challenges as opportunities for learning and growth. Single moms can teach themselves to embrace change, adapt to new circumstances, and continually develop new skills to thrive in any situation.

Seeking Professional Help When Needed:
Therapists, counselors, or life coaches can provide valuable guidance for managing stress, dealing with emotions, and making important

life decisions. Seeking professional help is a sign of strength and a step toward ensuring overall well-being.

Thriving as a single mom involves a combination of self-care, support systems, effective strategies, and a positive mindset. With determination, resourcefulness, and the willingness to learn and grow, single moms can navigate the challenges they face and create a fulfilling and prosperous life for themselves and their children. Remember, every achievement, big or small, is a testament to the strength of the single mom spirit.

Celebrating Milestones

Being a single mom comes with its unique set of challenges and responsibilities. However, it's important to recognize and celebrate the significant milestones achieved throughout this journey. From personal achievements to those of your children, each accomplishment deserves to be acknowledged and commemorated. Celebrating milestones as a single mom not only boosts self-esteem and resilience but also creates lasting memories for both you and your children.

Personal Achievements:
Single moms often juggle multiple roles, from parenting to providing financially and managing the household. Celebrate your personal achievements, whether it's completing a degree, excelling at work, or pursuing a hobby. These accomplishments demonstrate your strength, determination, and ability to overcome obstacles while setting a positive example for your children.

Child's Milestones:
Every milestone your child reaches is a moment of pride. Whether it's their first step, the first day of school, or achieving academic excellence, these moments reflect the love, care, and guidance you provide. Celebrate these milestones with enthusiasm, showing your child that you value their growth and development.

Building Traditions:
Creating special traditions around milestones can foster a sense of togetherness and anticipation. Whether it's a family outing, a special meal, or a small gift, these traditions become cherished memories that your children will carry into their adulthood.

Seeking Support:
Celebrate by reaching out to your support network. Friends and family can provide encouragement and share in your joy. Additionally, joining support groups for single parents can offer a sense of belonging and a platform to celebrate achievements and milestones collectively.

Self-Care Celebrations:
Taking care of yourself is crucial. Celebrate your milestones by indulging in self-care activities, such as a spa day, a weekend getaway, or even a quiet evening with a good book. Acknowledging

your accomplishments and treating yourself enhances your well-being and self-worth.

Documenting the Journey:
Keep a journal, scrapbook, or photo album to document both your personal achievements and your child's milestones. Reflecting on how far you've come can be incredibly empowering, and these records can serve as a source of inspiration during challenging times.

Teaching Resilience:
Celebrating milestones within the context of single motherhood teaches your children resilience and the importance of acknowledging progress, no matter the circumstances. It instills in them the values of hard work, determination, and the ability to find joy in life's achievements.

Celebrating milestones as a single mom is about recognizing the strength, love, and dedication you pour into your role. By embracing personal achievements, rejoicing in your child's growth, building traditions, seeking support, practicing self-care, and documenting the journey, you create a positive and uplifting environment for both yourself and your children. Each milestone is a testament to your resilience and the deep bond you share with your family, forming a tapestry of cherished memories that will endure for years to come.